Ten Amazing Things That **Community Health Workers** Do Well

SOPHIA C. LONDON Ph.D.
Certified Christian Counselor | Trauma-Informed Coach | CHW Instructor

ISBN: 979-8-9986012-0-0
Printed in the United States of America

DEDICATION

To every Community Health Worker — named or unnamed, trained or self-taught, certified or simply called — this book is for you.

This is for those who answer late-night calls, step out into rain, snow, or sweltering heat, not for recognition, but out of pure love for the work and for the people you serve. You move through neighborhoods, knock on doors, comfort the sick, uplift the tired, and listen — really listen — to voices that often go unheard. Regardless of race, language, background, or belief, you show up. Every single time.

You are the bridge between care and community, between despair and hope. You are the ones who form walking groups so neighbors feel supported. You help manage A1Cs, encourage health screenings, and create safe spaces for dialogue and healing. You are the spark that turns concern into action, isolation into connection, and health statistics into real-life change.

Many of you do this work without a title, without a paycheck that reflects your worth, and too often without the applause you deserve. Yet, you keep going. Because deep inside, there is a fire. A dream. A purpose. Some of you were born for this. Others stumbled into it and found your calling. But all of you make a difference that can't be measured in charts or degrees.

This is for those who lay their heads down at night with tired bodies but full hearts, knowing that today — even if just for one person — you were an angel. A lifeline. A reminder that someone cares.

And yes — keep growing. Keep learning. Keep pushing forward. The world needs you, in the community and beyond. Never doubt the dent you've already made in the world — and the many more still to come.

With all the respect and gratitude in my heart,

This book is dedicated to you.

CONTENTS

ACKNOWLEDGMENTS

To the God of creation who from the beginning of time knew that his daughter Sophia Clementina was going to be able to do more than she could see and expect or imagine. For saving my life so many times, and for loving me the way that he does…thank you!

To my Husband who has been an encourager, for the days I felt like all the work and effort did not make any sense thank you

To my heart

Princess Lisseth and Princess Lhorraine thank you for always being a loving critic of my work.

For my Prince who I hope to make proud

To my sister who we call the crazy one, she is so smart and amazing, thank you for always being there for me

To all the people who I asked to read this book when it really was unreadable because it was written in Spanglish, thank you so much for your patience dedication, and love.

To all of you, who will read this book, I hope that after reading this book, you will learn something that you did not know about yourself, that by having the courage to answer sincerely and privately you would honestly… Know Thyself.

FORWARD

Thirty years ago, I was a woman with big dreams but limited English, carrying nothing but hope and determination in my heart. I had just arrived in this new country, Panama behind me, a world of challenges ahead of me.

When I first came to the United States, everything was different. The language felt like a mountain I needed to climb, and the culture was so unfamiliar. But I was not alone. I had my family - my husband Jose, my two beautiful daughters, and the strength of generations of resilient women before me.

My great-grandmother from Calcutta and my great-grandfather from Jamaica had already shown me that boundaries are just illusions. They had crossed oceans, and survived challenges, and here I was, continuing that legacy of strength.

Working with immigrant families became more than a job - it became my calling. I understood their struggles intimately. I knew what it meant to not speak the language, to feel lost, to need help. So when I worked with families ensuring their children got vaccinations, or helping them understand the healthcare system, I was not just doing a job. I was giving back, with all the love and passion in my heart.

My motivation was simple: to create a better life for my loved ones and to help others do the same.

This is why I became a Community Health Worker. This is why I continue to serve.

CHAPTER 1

MY STORY

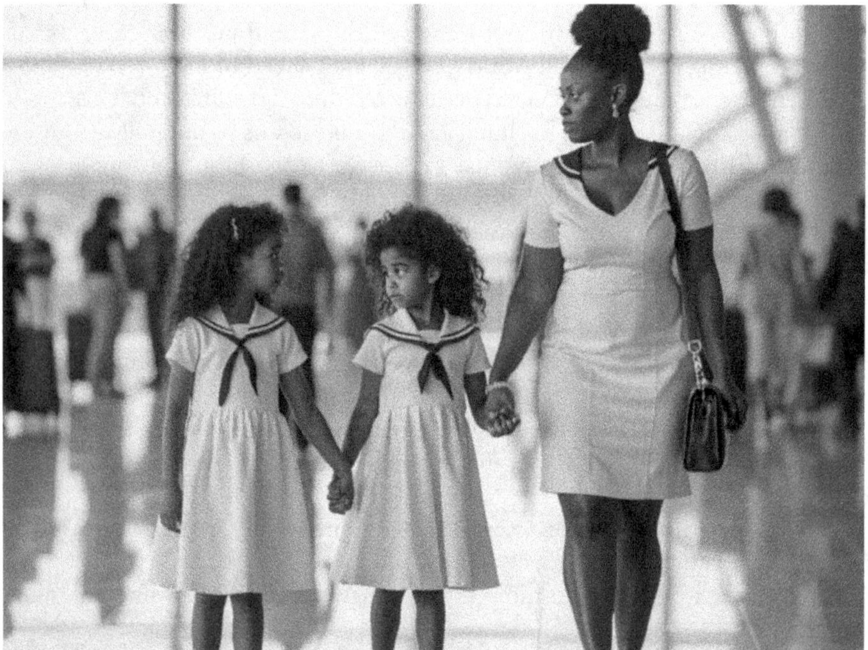

In August of 1995, I arrived at LaGuardia Airport with my two young daughters, ages seven and nine, not knowing what the future would hold for us. Like every foreigner who comes to this country hoping for a better future, that is what I wanted for my girls—the opportunity of a lifetime. I could not understand what was said, but I was excited for what the future had in store. We made it to New York, the beautiful New York that historically has been the transition point of so many stories like mine.

As I stood in that bustling airport, surrounded by the cacophony of languages and movement, my heart was a mixture of hope and uncertainty. My daughters clung close to me, their small hands gripping my own, their eyes wide with a combination of wonder and apprehension. We were strangers in a strange land, but we were together.

My happiness in New York quickly dissolved into pure frustration. The city was overwhelming - nothing like my beloved Panama. Everything moved at a pace so rapid, so chaotic, so different from the quiet, relaxed rhythm I had known my entire life. The language felt like a barrier, thick and impenetrable. There were moments I questioned everything - was this dream of a better life worth the struggle? Was I strong enough to continue?

But resilience runs deep in my blood. My family has always been my anchor, my compass. My sister in Minneapolis called and said, "Sophia, Minnesota will be better for you and the girls." She spoke with such conviction that I trusted her immediately. Most of my family had already settled in Minneapolis, which meant support, community, *familia.*

So, with determination in my heart and hope in my suitcases, I packed my daughters and we boarded the Greyhound bus heading to Minnesota. August in Minnesota was our first taste of cold - so different from Panama's warmth. But we were together, and that was what mattered most.

My sister welcomed us at the bus stop, her daughters surrounding us with familiar faces and love. We had not seen each other since Panama, and now here we were, starting a new chapter together. The moment felt both terrifying and beautiful.

Registering the girls in school became my priority. I wanted them to have every possible advantage, every tool for success. My sister who spoke perfect English accompanied me, helping me navigate the complicated registration process. My daughters would be in school with their cousins - a small comfort in a sea of uncertainty.

I knew their language barriers would be challenging, but I was determined to ensure they had accessible support. My girls were brave, and resilient - just like their mother. We would face this new world together, step by step, with love and determination.

English Language Advancement: The 2-Year Immersion

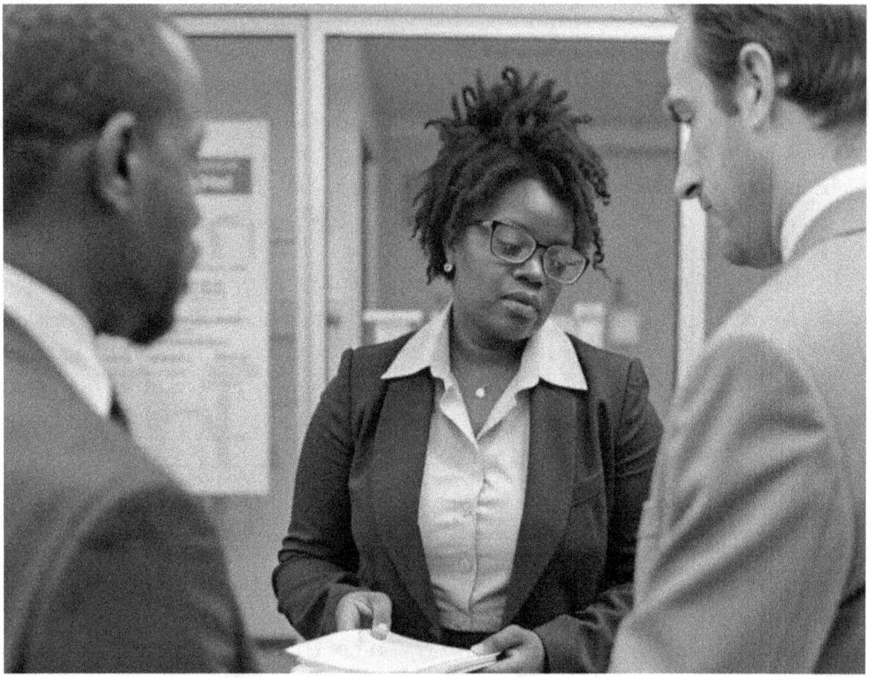

Navigating a new system in a foreign land was a monumental task, but I was determined to make it work for my family. I secured a job at a bank where my primary responsibilities were filing and copying documents. This position, although it didn't require me to speak English, became a classroom of sorts for me. Every day, I was surrounded by the hum of conversations, and I seized this opportunity to train my ears to the nuances of the English language. People spoke swiftly, their words initially a blur, but little by little, I began to pick out words, then phrases. It was a challenging process, but I was amazed at my gradual progress.

Our family routine became a well-oiled machine. My husband worked night shifts and took care of the girls in the morning, while I worked from 6 a.m. to 2:30 p.m., ensuring I was there to meet my daughters after school. This schedule was our backbone for many years, providing stability amidst the chaos of adapting to a new life.

However, life in the office wasn't without its struggles. I recall a day when my supervisor rushed into the room, delivered a message quickly, and left before I could grasp any of it. I felt lost and had to ask a coworker to repeat his message. It turned out we had an imminent staff meeting to discuss new work distribution changes. Sitting in that meeting, surrounded by fast-paced English, my frustration mounted—I understood nothing. Yet, I clung to my determination, ensuring that what I lacked in language skills, I made up for in the quality of my work.

As time passed, my understanding deepened. I started recognizing complete sentences and could keep up better with the speed of conversation. Eager to advance, I approached a temp agency for training. The first skill I tackled was using the ten-key by touch. The first skill I set my heart on mastering was using the ten-key by touch. This skill is crucial for anyone working in administrative roles, especially in fields like accounting and data entry, where speed and accuracy are paramount. The ten-key pad includes numbers 0 through 9, arranged to facilitate quick numeric input without the need to look at the keys.

Determined to enhance my job prospects, I found a large, second-hand calculator at a local thrift store—a humble but significant tool for my practice. Each night, after the day's chores and responsibilities, I devoted time to perfecting this skill. I would sit at our modest kitchen table, the calculator stationed before me, my fingers methodically tapping away. It was not just about pressing keys; it was about building muscle memory, training my fingers to know each key's location instinctively.

This practice became a nightly ritual, a quiet moment of focus and determination. With each correct sequence of numbers, my confidence grew. I was not merely learning a technical skill; I was paving a path to a better future, driven by the desire to provide more for my daughters and prove to myself that I could thrive in this new land. This dedication to mastering the ten-key by touch was a testament to my resolve, a small but significant triumph in my journey of personal and professional growth.

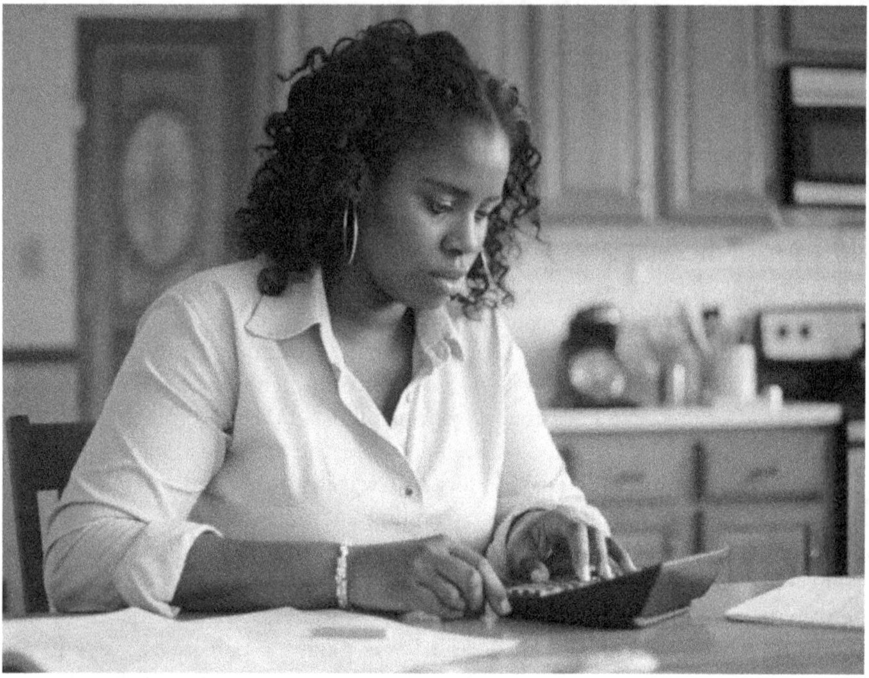

A month later, I informed the agency I was ready to test my speed, aiming for a better-paying job. No more was I content with just copying files for $6.50 an hour; I was ready to challenge myself further.

I then invested in a second-hand computer and taught myself to type. Understanding that better opportunities required not just language proficiency but also technical skills, I focused on improving my typing speed and accuracy. My efforts paid off, and within a year, I was earning $7.50 an hour—a respectable wage at the time.

My sister advised me, "Save your money, get your own place, my nieces deserve their own space." I rented my first apartment, bought furniture for my girls' bedroom, and moved out of my sister's apartment. I love her and am eternally grateful to her for her sound advice. She is gone from this world but still has a big space in my heart.

I met people who were willing to explain slowly what was said so I could be effective. This motivated me, when it was my turn to work with foreigners, to extend to them the same courtesy, patience, and respect I was given as a foreigner. I realized that many people I come in contact with today need the same help I needed when I came to this country, which includes empathy, understanding, patience, and compassion.

I am committed to serve everyone regardless of race, color, religion, creed, language, nationality, belief, or any differences. In my world, it does not matter, I serve.

Social & Literal Translations of the Heart

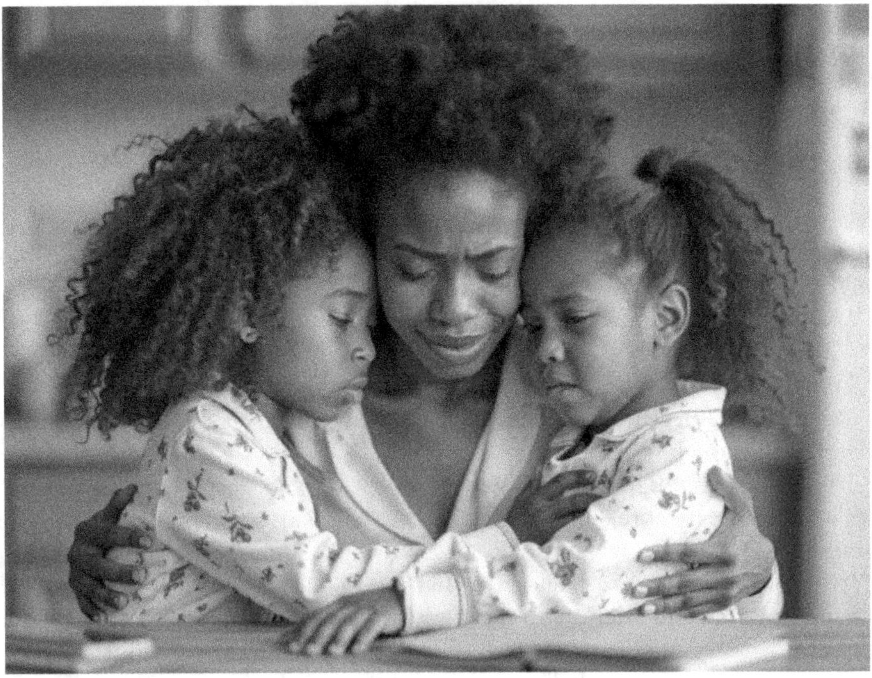

During my time working with Baby Tracks and Child & Teen Checkup, I found myself deeply embedded in the heart of various immigrant communities, including the Somali, Hmong, and Latino populations. My role, though unofficially titled at the time, mirrored that of Community Health Workers.

"I was doing the work of Community Health Workers without the title," I would often say.

It was a role I embraced with open arms as I loved the direct interaction and the opportunity to make a tangible difference in these communities.

Each day was filled with the responsibility of setting up tables in community centers and conducting presentations on vital health topics. I covered everything from the importance of using baby chairs correctly to the benefits of flu shots, smoking cessation, and how to conduct breast exams at home. This was vital information for these families, many of whom were navigating the complexities of a new healthcare system in a new country.

I was thriving in my job, I recall, reflecting on those busy, fulfilling days. However, alongside my professional successes, I encountered a personal challenge that brought a stark realization: the necessity of mastering English not just for myself, but crucially for my daughters.

One vivid memory that stands out was a visit to my daughter's school. I was eager to learn about their progress, but what I discovered instead led to a critical turning point.

When I learned that they were placed in a special classroom, I innocently asked, "Oh, great! What is so special about this classroom?"

The teacher's response was a jolt to my reality. "In this classroom, the kids cannot understand the teacher and vice versa," she explained.

My heart sank as I pressed further, "So when will they leave this classroom?" The teacher's sad look and her silent departure left me stunned and outraged.

"How rude, but how sad," I thought to myself.

That evening was a turning point. I returned home, heavy with thoughts on how to tackle this new hurdle. After praying for guidance, I had a serious conversation with my girls.

I said, "Babies, the teacher thinks you are dumb and stupid."

Their shocked expressions mirrored the gravity of the situation.

"Why, Mama?" they asked.

I explained, "Because you cannot understand the teacher. You don't speak English well enough to leave that classroom."

I told my girls, "Babies, this is what will happen: In this house, we will not speak Spanish anymore, and we will not watch Spanish programs on the television."

This conversation was a catalyst for change. It underscored the urgent need for us to improve our English skills, not just to thrive academically but to navigate our new world with confidence. This moment was not just about confronting a language barrier but about challenging the subtle prejudices that could hinder our progress. It motivated me even more to advocate for not only my children but also for the many families in the immigrant communities I worked with, ensuring they received the support and respect they deserved.

The raw emotions of that pivotal evening are etched deeply in my memory. Upon hearing the plan to banish Spanish from our home, my youngest, Princess Lho, voiced her confusion and hurt, "But we just came, why would she think that?"

Her words pierced me, reflecting the innocence and bewilderment of a child thrust too quickly into an unforgiving situation.

I gathered my girls close, the weight of my decision heavy on my shoulders as I explained, "Babies, this is what will happen: In this house, we will not speak Spanish anymore, and we will not watch Spanish programs on the television."

The look of disbelief in their eyes, the tears that started to form, broke my heart, but I held firm. I hugged them tightly, trying to offer comfort even as I imposed this harsh new rule. "I was as serious as a heart attack," I would later reflect, recognizing the gravity of my decision.

The following months were some of the most challenging in our lives. The girls, stripped of the comfort of their mother tongue at home, faced the daunting task of immersing themselves completely in English. It was a drastic measure, one that pained me deeply. I literally traumatized my daughters to accomplish this–I admit–not without a sense of regret for the emotional toll it took on them.

However, the results were undeniable. Within three months, they had transitioned out of the special education classroom, a testament to their resilience and adaptability.

As for me, my journey with the English language was far more tortuous. Despite my best efforts, I did not learn English as efficiently or as quickly as my daughters did. This created a new set of challenges, particularly when it came to helping them with their homework. "My verbs were non-existent, and I felt like I was a mess," I recall, the frustration palpable even now.

For me, learning English was not merely about adapting to a new country—it was a survival tool, an essential bridge for my daughters and me to cross into a world of better opportunities. My journey with the English language was filled with both missteps and milestones. I remember vividly one family movie night that turned into a humorous, yet eye-opening experience. "I chose an action movie for the family to watch, thinking I knew enough English by then," I recall. The movie was *Long Kiss Goodnight* with Geena Davis and Samuel Jackson. But oh, within the first ten minutes, Samuel Jackson's character was cursing like a sailor. "We did not finish the movie," I chuckle now, remembering the switch to a cartoon instead. "To let you know how bad my comprehension was, I didn't even know he was cursing."

This incident, though lighthearted, underscored a serious challenge. It was a stark reminder of the language barriers that still existed for us.

As a mother, seeing my daughters face similar challenges was tough. When my eldest, Princess Li, was in middle school, a comment from her principal left me both hurt and furious. "She may need to settle her goals of working in a store as a cashier because she is slow," he said. I had to put on a fake smile, defending her by explaining, "She thinks in Spanish. The time you think she is being slow, she is translating the words in her mind."

The realization that Princess Li was advancing through grades without being able to read was a shock that propelled me into action. This was unacceptable. Without reading, there would be no college. Without college, no professional career. Without reading, no professional excellence. At least that is what I believed then—not now, but that is a story for another time.

I confronted the school principal, insisting, "Princess Li cannot read. You need to fix it." It was a pivotal moment, leading to a change in teachers and a renewed focus on her literacy.

Thanks to the relentless efforts of a dedicated teacher who took my concerns seriously, Princess Li not only learned to read but excelled beyond expectations. "She graduated, went on to get her bachelor's degree, then her master's, and then her PhD," I say with immense pride. She is now an international trauma-informed psychologist, a testament to the power of determination and the right educational support.

With my youngest, Princess Lho, the challenges were different but equally daunting. As she neared high school graduation, she expressed a desire to attend college in New York. The very thought filled me with fear—fear of losing her to a vast, overwhelming city. "I had to use the phrase my parents used on me," I confess. "I don't want you with her or him," I told her, deciding instead that she would go to college in Nebraska. Though she never forgave me for that decision, it gave me peace of mind. Today, she holds two master's degrees, an MBA, a PMP, and runs her own successful business.

Reflecting on these experiences, I see a tapestry of struggle, resilience, and ultimate triumph woven by the hands of a mother determined to ensure her daughters' success. "It takes a whole family and caring teachers to make a difference," I often say, acknowledging that our journey was a collective effort. Our story is a testament to the power of perseverance, the importance of education, and the unyielding love of a mother for her children. It is these values I hope to pass on through my work and my writing, inspiring others to overcome their barriers and reach for their dreams.

These experiences, though fraught with difficulty and emotional strain, were foundational. They not only shaped our family's path forward but also deepened my commitment to my work with immigrant families. Understanding firsthand the barriers language can create; I was even more driven to advocate for and support those navigating similar challenges. This period of our lives, while marked by trials, ultimately fortified our resolve and united us in our journey toward a better future.

Now I need you to understand that the only reason I told you part of my story is for you to know that leaving your country was the first step to accepting that we are ready to make positive changes in our lives. Working hard and looking at each challenge straight on, knowing that this will make you stronger, better, and a great example for your loved ones, is the key to this book.

I also want to mention that I found many people who believe that because you are not a foreigner, this book is not for you. I do want to remind you what my professor drilled in my head when I was beating myself up because I could not grasp English fast enough. He said, "Your ancestors had to adapt, learn, and suffer, and they made it." I remember saying, "No sir, my ancestors are not from here, they are from Panama." He smiled and said, "Even in your country, if your people were not Indian, then they were foreigners." He smiled and told me I was going to be okay in time, and not to stop learning and trying to be better.

To you, I say, someone in your family paid the price for you to be where and who you are today. Embrace it, respect it, and if you can, pay it forward!

If and when you ever come into a new country, leaving all you have known—friends, neighbors, teachers, classmates, and people you grew up with grandparents, or in many cases even your own parents—know that it is a very hard thing to do. So put in the effort to make the sacrifice worth all that you left behind by never settling for less or giving up. Making the best out of that sacrifice is the key.

In the next few pages, you will discover the valuable contributions of Community Health Workers (CHWs). Like any profession, you will find that some are well-trained, while others are in the process of upgrading their skills and resources. However, their primary goal remains to help and serve the community. These skilled professionals are always learning to better serve those in need.

CHWs come from diverse backgrounds, encompassing various colors, races, shapes, languages, religions, and denominations. Despite these differences, their dedication to service is their common driving force.

These professionals possess a unique ability to observe what is not immediately apparent, listen to what is unsaid, and understand circumstances without judgment or prejudice. They utilize all available resources to ensure they provide the highest quality, efficiency, effectiveness, and support to those who need help.

There are many professions in the world. Some people are fortunate enough to do what they love, while others do what they must to survive. If you ever feel inferior compared to doctors, attorneys, judges, teachers, firefighters, police officers, mechanics, barbers, beauticians, secretaries, receptionists, social workers, or any other respected professions, remember that you are valuable. If you love what you do and make a difference in someone's life, that makes you valuable.

There is a famous actor (Ken Jeong) who initially trained as a surgeon, fulfilling his family's expectations. However, his true passion was acting. Despite his family's skepticism, he pursued his dream and is now a successful and happy actor. The lesson here is to be efficient in whatever you do, and when you find your true passion, work hard to be successful and enjoy every minute of it.

Over time, many of us realize that giving is better than receiving, and at that moment of realization, we take great joy in giving back, blessing others, and improving someone's life. It's a natural progression in life.

Regardless of your career choice, if you aim to be a Community Health Worker (CHW), you must genuinely love, not just like, dealing with all kinds of people. You'll encounter individuals who are rude, disrespectful, loud, noisy, shy, educated, uneducated, calm, rambunctious, dishonest, proud, silent, scared, and sometimes dangerous. Understand that many may never repay you or even say thank you. Some you may help once and never see again. Knowing this truth motivates CHWs to provide quality and efficient care the first time because they may never have another opportunity to help that person again.

Community Health Worker (CHW) programs are a cornerstone of public health in both low- and middle-income countries (LMICs) and high-income countries (HICs). From the bustling streets of **India and Brazil** to the remote villages of **Malawi and Nepal**, CHWs are delivering frontline healthcare, education, and hope.

CHWs are making a significant impact in countries such as: **Afghanistan, Bangladesh, Brazil, Ethiopia, India, Indonesia, Iran, Liberia, Malawi, Nepal, Niger, Rwanda, Zambia, Zimbabwe, Kenya, Tanzania, Mali, Uganda, Sierra Leone, and Ghana.**

Organizations like **UNICEF** highlight the essential work of female CHWs in countries including **Nepal, Ecuador, Afghanistan, and Nigeria**, while **Orb Media** provides a global overview of their roles in nations such as **Hungary,**

Chile, and Thailand.

As of 2024, it is estimated that **4.7 million CHWs** are serving worldwide, based on reports from **100 countries**, though 71% of the reported data comes from the years **2019–2023**, suggesting the real number may be even higher.

CHWs continue to be the hands and feet of healthcare—bridging gaps, saving lives, and transforming communities one visit at a time.

TEN AMAZING THINGS CHWS DO BEST

1. **Listening:** Beyond hearing, CHWs listen to unspoken words, analyze short phrases loaded with information, observe body language, and evaluate surroundings for safety. They listen to bring solutions, not just answers.
2. **Dress Well and Maintain Self-Care**: Maintaining a professional appearance and personal well-being is essential.
3. **Know Your Boundaries:** CHWs understand their limits and act accordingly.
4. **Act Appropriately:** They adjust their behavior depending on the situation and the people involved.
5. **Recognize Bias:** CHWs are aware of and actively combat bias.
6. **Speak to All:** They communicate effectively with everyone, regardless of social or intellectual status.
7. **Door-to-Door Outreach:** CHWs often visit homes to provide essential services like food pantries and health screenings.
8. **Stay Educated:** They remain knowledgeable and up-to-date within their field.
9. **Understand Immigration:** CHWs are informed about immigration issues that may affect their clients.
10. **Respect Themselves and Their Career:** They maintain self-respect and take pride in their profession.

LISTENING: A KEY SKILL OF CHWS

Listening is a fundamental skill for CHWs. It involves not just hearing but truly understanding what is being communicated, both verbally and non-verbally. For example, I met Angelica at a barbershop where I was announcing the opening of a clinic for undocumented individuals, the working poor, and those without insurance. Angelica approached me as I was leaving, and although she appeared calm, her words indicated she was in danger. She confessed to stabbing her husband in self-defense after he beat her.

Despite my initial urge to panic, I remained calm and assessed the situation. I suggested calling an ambulance for her husband. Angelica provided the address, and just then, her brother-in-law emerged. Seeing her distress, he understood something was wrong. We explained the situation, and he took her to the house where the ambulance was already attending to her husband. It turned out that her husband had been caught with her best friend, leading to a violent altercation.

By staying calm and attentive, I helped ensure her husband received medical attention, preventing a potential tragedy. This incident underscores the importance of listening, observing body language and remaining composed under pressure. With proper training, CHWs can handle such situations effectively, providing vital support and potentially saving lives.

DRESSING WELL AND MAINTAINING SELF-CARE

As a Community Health Worker (CHW), presenting yourself professionally is crucial. I once attended a meeting where I felt uncomfortable because a man couldn't stop staring at my chest. I realized that by not dressing appropriately, I had inadvertently drawn unwanted attention to myself. This taught me the importance of dressing modestly and professionally for work.

When you are out in the field, such as at a food pantry, it's important not to draw attention with revealing clothing, tattoos, or inappropriate attire. You're there to help and support the community, not to stand out. For instance, I once worked alongside a lady who wore excessive jewelry and party makeup at a school outreach event. It was clear she wasn't dressed for the occasion.

Dressing Tips for Community Health Workers:

- **Modesty:** Choose clothing that covers appropriately. Avoid low-cut tops or anything too tight.
- **Professionalism:** Wear simple, clean, and appropriate attire.
- **Occasion:** Dress according to the event you're attending—no party outfits for work events.

You might think, "Everyone knows this," but you'd be surprised how many don't consider it.

Self-Care

Self-care is another critical aspect of being an effective CHW. The job's demands can be overwhelming, and it's important to take care of yourself to provide the best care to others.

Imagine you came home late from a mammogram outreach, had to prepare dinner, help the kids with homework, and then found out your daughter, Perla, needed 75 cupcakes for school the next day. You stay up late baking, and the next day at the food pantry, your patience runs thin. Clients start getting on your nerves with specific requests, and in a moment of frustration, you snap and say, "This is why I hate working with you people. Always taking and taking and don't even deserve it!"

The Importance of Self-Care:

- **Know Your Limits:** Understand when you're not at your best and take time out.
- **Rest and Rejuvenate:** Ensure you get enough rest and time for yourself.
- **Permission to Pause:** If you encounter a particularly tough situation, take a break. My supervisor once told us we could take time off if a story or incident shook us up. Serving less than 95% of your capacity affects not only you but also your clients.

Self-care is not just for your benefit; it impacts everyone around you. Love yourself enough to take the necessary steps to maintain your well-being, and everyone will be grateful.

In Summary

Dressing well and self-care are fundamental to being a successful Community Health Worker. Present yourself professionally to avoid unwanted attention and distractions. Prioritize self-care to ensure you can provide the best support to your clients. When you care for yourself, you're better equipped to care for others.

KNOW YOUR BOUNDARIES

Oh my, I could talk about this for hours. I come from a generation that enforced certain boundaries: do not interrupt adults while they speak, leave the room when adults are talking, chew with your mouth closed, and never roll your eyes.

However, when it comes to community work, boundaries need to be even more stringent. Consider Isabella, who was working with a client whose A1C level was 12. To help manage this condition, Isabella connected with the client twice a month, both over the phone and face-to-face. Isabella maintained clear boundaries initially, but the client began to overstep, calling Isabella her friend, sharing personal household issues, and contacting her frequently, even on weekends. Their face-to-face meetings turned into lunch dates with the client paying for meals, and Isabella started accepting small gifts. This inappropriate relationship escalated until the client's husband accused Isabella of dating his wife and lodged an official complaint, leading to Isabella's suspension without pay pending an investigation.

In your opinion, was it justified to suspend Isabella? Yes, it was. Although the situation may have begun innocently, Isabella's failure to enforce professional boundaries led to a serious ethical breach.

The Importance of Boundaries

Boundaries are crucial for maintaining professionalism and integrity in community health work. Here's why:

- **Protects Professional Relationships:** Boundaries ensure that relationships with clients remain professional and do not cross into personal territories.
- **Maintains Objectivity:** By keeping interactions professional, CHWs can provide unbiased, effective care.
- **Prevents Misunderstandings:** Clear boundaries prevent situations where actions can be misinterpreted, as happened with Isabella.
- **Ensures Accountability:** Boundaries hold both the CHW and the

client accountable to professional standards.

Setting Boundaries in Community Health Work:

- **Clear Communication:** Define your availability and stick to it. Explain to clients the appropriate times and ways to contact you.
- **Professional Interactions:** Keep all interactions, whether over the phone or in person, professional. Avoid meeting in social settings like restaurants or accepting gifts.
- **Consistent Enforcement:** If a client oversteps boundaries, gently but firmly remind them of your professional guidelines.
- **Seek Guidance:** If you are unsure about a situation, seek advice from a supervisor or a colleague to ensure you are handling it appropriately.

Conclusion

Boundaries are essential for being honest, reliable, efficient, effective, and flexible. They protect you, your clients, and your professional license. Remember, maintaining boundaries is not just a part of your job; it is crucial to your success and integrity as a Community Health Worker. You are the embodiment of these boundaries.

ACT ACCORDINGLY

Community Health Workers (CHWs) can work in various settings under the supervision of doctors, attorneys, dentists, clinics, community centers, or other agencies focused on patient and client well-being.

For instance, Yadira worked with Shanirra, a nurse practitioner at a dentist's office. Upon arrival, Yadira asked Shanirra what she needed from her that day. Shanirra outlined the patients needing extra attention, detailed the paperwork process, and explained how to break down the questions on the forms. She also instructed Yadira to ensure the mammogram technicians received water and lunch. Thanks to clear communication and understanding of roles, the day was successful. Twenty-five of the 35 expected clients were seen, forms were correctly filled out, clients understood what they were signing, and technicians received their meals.

Understanding and Accepting Your Role

Being a CHW is one of the most rewarding careers, offering the choice to work in an office, in the community, or a combination of both. It's crucial to know, understand, and accept your role and tasks for the day.

For example, Malory, a CHW with a community center program, invited a nurse to check attendees' blood sugar and blood pressure. Malory mingled with the attendees, encouraging them to get checked, which contributed to the program's success. This demonstrates the importance of knowing your place and task.

The Importance of Professional Conduct

On the other hand, consider Danny, a practitioner who doesn't speak Spanish, and Marielena, who was asked to interpret for him. Instead of sticking to her role, Marielena added her own experiences and jokes, which Danny did not understand. **If you were Danny, how would that make you feel?**

Danny would likely feel frustrated and undermined. Marielena's behavior could lead to miscommunication, reduce the professionalism of the interaction, and potentially cause misunderstandings with the clients.

Key Points for Acting Accordingly:

- **Know Your Role:** Clearly understand your duties for the day.
- **Respect Boundaries:** Stick to your tasks without overstepping others' responsibilities.
- **Professional Conduct:** Maintain professionalism in all interactions.
- **Effective Communication:** Ensure clear, respectful communication with supervisors and colleagues.

Conclusion

Community Health Workers are task-oriented and adapt their roles depending on the program and who is in charge. Acting accordingly means understanding and respecting your role, maintaining professionalism, and ensuring effective communication. By doing so, CHWs contribute to the success of their programs and provide the best possible support to their clients.

RECOGNIZE BIAS

I grew up with grandparents who were light-skinned compared to me, and with family members who didn't like Black people. We had slang for Black people, Asians, and White people. Kids in school can be mean, although thankfully, not all of them are... or are they?

To be efficient and effective, you need to be honest about your biases. I have issues working with anyone who beats their spouse. I can work with people of any race, religion, or denomination, but not with abusers. I have not built up the courage to love them unconditionally...yet!

What about you? ______________________________________

Who are you not able to work with and why? ____________________
____
____
____

If you find it difficult to work with a particular type of person or group of people, which one is it and why? ___________________________
____
____
____

Understanding your limitations can help you identify the audience that can benefit from your work.

Personal Story

My father beat my mother like she was a man or a rag doll. He would punch as strongly as he could as if he were punching a man. One time they were having a good day, and he started wrestling with her. She accidentally knocked him out cold. When he woke up, he hit her with a chair across her back. She ended up in the ER, and after that day, there were no more friendly wrestling matches.

Working with Bias

I worked at the bus station helping migrants buy tickets, explaining their routes, and how many times the Greyhound bus would stop. One day, I helped a group of migrants. They took their bus, and I gave them food and blankets for the journey. One man stood there watching me help others. Despite my offers of drinks, food, and snacks, he always responded with "nothing" (Nada, no puedes hacer nada por mí).

My shift was ending, so I approached him, determined to help. I said "Sir, I have watched you for more than two hours, I asked you on many occasions if you needed anything, but your answer was always the same, no you cannot help me. Sir. That is not true, I am leaving in 30 minutes, how can I help you" He looked at me, his face this time looking less stern and hard, and he said, " I was told not to trust Black people." My heart broke. He was so hurt, scared, and in need, but what he had been told was stronger than his fear and need.

I explained to him that years ago, I was in his position. I arrived in a foreign country with two daughters, speaking a different language. I was scared but had to be strong, courageous, and bold for my girls. I had to accept help from strangers because I needed it. Today, I give back because I know what it feels like. So, I asked him again, "What can I do for you?" He replied, "I have watched you, and you do not look like what they told me."

It was the end of my shift, so we helped him buy a ticket to his destination, put him up in a hotel for the night, and promised to pick him up the next day. We sent him off with water, food, blankets, and snacks for the road. That day, my boundaries fell, and we hugged. He cried, and I gave him my number and promised that if he called me, I would connect him to CHW in the city he was going to, ensuring he would get help, even if the helper's skin color was one he initially distrusted.

Conclusion

If you are prejudiced or secretly biased, you cannot effectively help others, improve lives, or help yourself grow. The world needs your God-given talent to bless and heal.

Are you racist or prejudiced? The world needs you to overcome these biases to use your talents for the greater good.

Only you can answer that question and only you can decide how much and who you will be able to serve.

THE ART OF SPEAKING

I went into the neighborhood to talk about the impact of sugar and salt on our health. The PowerPoint presentation was clear, direct, and to the point. I explained why rice can make us sick and how salt can be harmful. I also discussed how our ancestors managed to stay healthy despite eating a lot of rice and salt—they walked everywhere.

After the talk, a lady approached me and asked if I could speak to her husband. Despite doctors warning him about his pre-diabetes, he still didn't understand the seriousness. This highlights that clarity in communication goes beyond just speaking English or Spanish; it's about using the right words for the right audience.

The Responsibility of Communication

Community Health Workers (CHWs) have the responsibility to effectively communicate with a wide range of people, for example: company presidents, managers, coworkers, clients, patients, and community members. Speaking is an art, and to master it, Community Health Workers need to tailor their communication to each and specific audience to ensure they receive and understand the correct information.

Tips for Effective Communication

1. **Avoid Talking Down to People**: Many people can speak a language but might struggle with reading or writing it, or vice versa. Don't assume everyone understands things the same way.
2. **Be Aware of Language Barriers**: Accents, different languages, or medical conditions like strokes can hinder communication. If you can't understand a client, professionally hand over the case to someone who can assist them better.
3. **Know Your Audience**: Use words and examples that resonate with your audience's experiences and knowledge levels.
4. **Practice Active Listening**: Ensure clients feel heard and understood. Clarify any misunderstandings and confirm their doubts and questions are

clear before they leave your presence.

Example of Ineffective Communication

I once knew a lady with two master's degrees who was a terrible communicator. She made college students feel foolish, and her tone was often rude and disrespectful. Despite her knowledge and skills, she was eventually fired due to her poor communication style and disrespectful body language.

Conclusion

If you cannot communicate effectively, you cannot help, change lives, or bless someone in desperate need. Be ready to be a blessing by being clear, listening actively, and ensuring clients leave knowing they were understood and served.

KNOW YOUR STRENGTHS AND WEAKNESSES

Community Health Workers (CHWs) have the ability to perform at the highest level of their skills. They excel in various settings, such as food pantries, mammogram outreaches, Flu shot clinics, and back-to-school events. translation, community centers. and more. Their role often involves communicating with clients, patients, community members, identifying additional needs, and providing holistic support, sometimes their major role is listening without judgment and giving comfort, and ensuring they know they are cared for.

The Role of a CHW in Different Settings

1. **Food Pantries**: CHWs interact with clients not only to distribute food but also to assess other needs. They walk from car to car, asking about additional requirements like medical appointments, dental care, or household items.

   Example: Patrick came to a food pantry for food. When asked about other needs, he revealed that he and his family were sleeping on the floor and needed basic household items. Through conversation, it became clear that Patrick also needed emotional support, the Community Health Workers continued to talk and listen to what Patrick was not saying. He was struggling in his current job, but could not, nor wanted to tell his wife about it to not stress her out. This highlights one of the crucial roles of the CHWs.
2. **Mammogram Outreach**: CHWs talk to attendees to determine if there are other health concerns or services they might need, ensuring a thorough approach to community health.
3. **Community Outreach**: CHWs engage with the community to understand broader needs, providing resources and connecting people with appropriate services.

Effective Communication and Emotional Support

A CHW must be trained to recognize and respond appropriately to the emotional states and needs of clients. This involves knowing when to listen more and when to provide more information.

Example: Patrick expressed deep emotional distress about his situation, which he couldn't share at home. The CHW provided a confidential space for him to express his feelings and assured him that his needs would be met, demonstrating the importance of empathy and support.

Handling Difficult Situations

CHWs often face challenging interactions and must remain patient and professional.

Example: When a woman complained rudely about not receiving a washing machine, the CHW handled the situation by finding out what happened to the request. She found out that there was no truck to deliver the machines the church had donated. The CHW called a friend and asked if he could deliver the machines and bring someone to help. The client could not lift them or help with that task. She went back to let the lady know that the machines would be delivered in the evening, explained to her what the problem was, and let her know that sometimes the church donated but transportation and delivery happen when members of the church are available to drop off the merchandise on the weekends, but there were too many deliveries for the group, that is why hers had to wait. The client was excited, calm, and understood the situation. By ensuring the machine would be delivered, the CHW maintained professionalism and ensured the client's needs were met despite the client's initial hostility.

Maintaining Professionalism

CHWs must uphold their reputation by delivering services with excellence, efficiency, and reliability as much as possible.

1. **Consistency**: Ensure that promises made to clients are kept and follow up on any issues that arise.
2. **Patience**: Understand that clients may be frustrated or angry due to their situations. Handling these emotions calmly is crucial.
3. **Empathy**: Recognize and respond to the emotional and practical needs of clients.

Conclusion

CHWs are vital in bridging gaps in healthcare and social services within communities. Their ability to communicate effectively, provide emotional support, and handle difficult situations with patience and professionalism makes them indispensable. Understanding and utilizing their strengths while acknowledging and addressing weaknesses ensures they can serve their communities with excellence and compassion.

EDUCATION FOR COMMUNITY HEALTH WORKERS

It is true that Community Health Workers (CHWs) often start with a certificate, but the value and impact of their work extend far beyond formal education. Here's why CHWs, even with just a certificate, are so effective in their roles:

Learning by Doing: The Power of Practical Skills

Much like mechanics who learn from each other, or individuals who gain practical skills by watching and helping others, CHWs also benefit from hands-on experience and learning from their community.

- **Practical Experience**: Just as someone might learn to fix a car by observing a mechanic, CHWs gain invaluable experience by working directly within their communities. They understand the specific needs and challenges their clients face and develop practical solutions.
- **Resourcefulness**: CHWs, like those who repair their homes or create handmade items, become resourceful problem-solvers. They learn to navigate the complex landscape of social services and healthcare resources to best serve their clients.

Networking and Community Connections

One of the most critical aspects of a CHW's education is building a network of contacts within the community. This network extends its ability to provide comprehensive support.

- **Community Resources**: CHWs must be knowledgeable about every resource available in their community, from utility assistance programs to housing information and healthcare services.
- **Establishing Connections**: Forming relationships with local businesses and agencies is crucial. CHWs connect with barbershops, beauty salons, restaurants, corner stores, second-hand shops, and other helpful connections to ensure they have a wide array of resources to offer their

clients.

- **Networking**: They also network with clinics, dentists, landlords, and other service providers, ensuring they can refer clients to the right place for their needs.

Continuous Learning and Professional Development

While a certificate provides a foundational knowledge base, continuous education is essential for CHWs to stay effective and up-to-date.

- **Ongoing Training**: Attending as many training sessions as possible helps CHWs stay current with the latest information and best practices. This continuous learning enhances their skills and effectiveness in the field.
- **Professional Growth**: Although many CHWs start with a certificate, they have opportunities to pursue further education, such as bachelor's, master's, and even doctoral degrees. However, even without advanced degrees, the hands-on training and practical knowledge they acquire are invaluable.

The Comprehensive Role of a CHW

The role of a CHW is multifaceted and extends beyond traditional classroom education. Their responsibilities include:

- **Information Gathering**: CHWs are often the first point of contact for clients needing various services. They gather detailed information about their clients' needs and connect them with appropriate resources.
- **Advocacy**: CHWs advocate for their clients, ensuring they receive the services they need and deserve, for example meeting their clients at doctor offices, or agencies to help them resolve their situation.
- **Community Liaison**: They act as a bridge between the community and health or social service providers, facilitating better understanding and cooperation.

Conclusion

Community Health Workers are equipped with a unique blend of formal education and practical, on-the-job learning. Their effectiveness lies in their ability to build strong community connections, continuously expand their knowledge through training, and apply practical solutions to real-world problems. By leveraging both formal education and experiential learning, CHWs play an essential role in enhancing the health and well-being of their communities.

IMMIGRATION: A CALL TO COMPASSION AND UNDERSTANDING

The experience of immigration is deeply complex and fraught with challenges that many cannot fully grasp without personal experience. Countries like the United States, Germany, Saudi Arabia, Russia, and the United Kingdom are witnessing a significant influx of migrants, and understanding their struggles and motivations is crucial for those who seek to help.

The Immigrant Experience

For many, leaving their homeland is not a choice but a necessity driven by the pursuit of safety, opportunity, and a better future for their families. The trauma of leaving loved ones, familiar surroundings, and a known way of life cannot be understated. It's essential to appreciate the gravity of their circumstances and the courage it takes to embark on such a journey.

Misconceptions and Realities

Television and media often paint a rosy picture of life in countries like the United States, suggesting that wealth and comfort are easily attainable. This misconception can lead to misunderstandings about the true struggles immigrants face upon arrival. For instance, seeing seemingly well-off individuals at food pantries might be perplexing to some, but it's important to recognize the hidden hardships and economic struggles many face,

Contributions and Sacrifices

Migrants play a vital role in the economy, often taking on jobs that are essential yet undervalued. Many undocumented workers contribute to the economy without the benefits of tax returns or job security. Their sacrifices extend beyond their immediate surroundings as they often send remittances back home, supporting families and communities they left behind.

Working with Immigrants: Essential Qualities

Heart and Compassion: Serving immigrants requires a deep sense of empathy and compassion. Understanding their journey and the trauma they have endured is fundamental to offering meaningful support.

Patience and Understanding: Immigrants are often navigating new systems, languages, and cultures. Patience is key in helping them understand their new environment and the resources available to them.

Non-Judgmental Attitude: It's essential to approach every immigrant without judgment. Their reasons for migrating are varied and personal, and respecting their experiences and choices is paramount.

Skills and Knowledge: Community Health Workers (CHWs) need to be well-informed about the resources available to immigrants. This includes legal aid, healthcare, housing, and employment services. Being a reliable source of information and guidance can significantly ease the transition for immigrants.

Stories of Struggle and Resilience

Hearing firsthand accounts from immigrants highlights the extreme difficulties they face. For example, Irma's journey through the jungle between Colombia and Panama, where she witnessed a friend fall victim to a crocodile, underscores the perilous paths many take to seek a better life. Such stories are sobering reminders of the dangers and desperation that drive migration.

The Role of Community Health Workers

CHWs are in a unique position to make a profound impact on the lives of immigrants. By providing support that preserves their dignity and respects their humanity, CHWs help restore a sense of hope and stability. The goal is to ensure that every interaction leaves the immigrant feeling respected, valued, and understood.

Conclusion

Working with immigrants is not just a job; it's a calling that demands compassion, patience, understanding, and dedication. By recognizing the immense challenges immigrants face and offering support with empathy and respect, Community Health Workers can play a crucial role in helping them build new lives with dignity and hope

RESPECT

Everyone has issues and traumas that live within them. Some are evident, while others are hidden. Take, for example, the little girl who just discovered that her father is not her biological father, that he was cruel to her mother, and that he was a wicked man. She also learns that she looks just like him. This revelation triggers her to start wetting the bed. No one knows how life will affect them. If you were not loved and cared for properly, you might misconstrue gentle and kind words as love, or if your first love cheated on you, you might punish every subsequent partner.

Life throws curveballs at us, and if we don't have a good head on our shoulders, we can make serious mistakes. Community Health Workers (CHWs) are particularly vulnerable to misinterpreting kindness as romantic interest.

Consider Veronica and Saul. Saul, a migrant from Venezuela, came to the US by crossing the border. Veronica helped him fill out his refugee paperwork and assisted him in finding jobs, first at a fast food restaurant and then at a mechanic shop where he excelled due to his background as a mechanic. They met for dinner one night because his busy schedule didn't allow for breakfast or lunch meetings. One thing led to another, and they started dating. Over time, Saul stopped talking about bringing his wife and two kids because he was now with Veronica.

You might think there's nothing wrong with this—just two people falling in love. But eight months later, his wife and two kids crossed the border and were detained for a while. When they were released, they found Saul, who then left Veronica to reunite with his family. The wife accused Veronica of luring her husband when he was lonely, scared, and desperate for help, claiming Veronica forced him to stay with her in exchange for her assistance.

CHWs must understand and recognize the importance of professionalism, maintaining boundaries, and self-respect. They help people from various backgrounds, including different countries, races, religions, languages, and beliefs. CHWs must be clear about their morals, mission, and vision to avoid damaging their reputation.

Respecting yourself means maintaining professional boundaries and steering clear of anything that feels dangerous or compromising.

For instance, Felipe runs a food pantry every Friday, ensuring families have enough groceries for the weekend. Latania, who volunteers at the pantry, has tried multiple times to flirt with Felipe, hoping for special treatment. Felipe constantly reminds her that every volunteer gets what they need and that dating him won't get her more. Her persistence led to the pastor intervening.

Respecting yourself means that your "no" means no, and your "yes" means yes. It involves articulating your words clearly, leaving no room for misinterpretation. CHWs must use precise language to ensure respect for themselves and others.

CHW EFFECTIVENESS

In my opinion, the following are the most important to ensure satisfaction and effectiveness:

CHWs in many countries are making a significant difference in the lives of diverse families, including single mothers or fathers, grandparents raising children, children raising siblings, and other family dynamics. These CHWs are working tirelessly in cities and towns, striving to improve lives and foster positive changes.

Below are some questions you need to answer sincerely. No one will correct or check your answers, but to help you grow and improve, these questions must be answered in the privacy of your own space, mind, and heart.

These questions will delve deeply into your soul. Remember, these are your life, your soul, and your personal answers:

1. Why did I choose to become a Community Health Worker?

   ____

   ____

   ____

   ____

2. What values and principles guide my work?

   ____

   ____

   ____

   ____

3. How do I handle personal boundaries in professional relationships?

   ____

   ____

   ____

   ____

4. Am I able to recognize when I am becoming too emotionally involved with a client?

5. What strategies do I use to maintain my professionalism in challenging situations?

6. Do I respect my own needs and limits as much as I respect those of my clients?

7. How do I ensure clear and respectful communication with the people I serve?

8. What do I do to continually improve my skills and knowledge as a CHW?

9. How do I deal with stress and prevent burnout in my role?

10. In what ways do I contribute to the community beyond my immediate responsibilities?

WHO ARE YOU?

Reflecting on these questions will help you become a more effective, compassionate, and professional Community Health Worker. Remember, the journey to self-improvement is ongoing, and your commitment to this process will benefit not only you but also the many lives you touch through your work.

1. Do you like yourself, and your character if not what you don't like?
   ____
   ____
   ____
   ____
2. Do you respect yourself, if not who hurt you so deeply that you don't respect yourself?
   ____
   ____
   ____
   ____
3. Do you like what you do, if not what is your dream job?
   ____
   ____
   ____
   ____
4. What race or color of people do you prefer to work with, and why?
   ____
   ____
   ____
   ____
5. Do you mean what you say, and keep promises most of the time, if not what is the problem and how can you improve that?
   ____

6. Is there any religious denomination or group of people you prefer not to work with, and why?

7. Do you respect single mothers or not really, and if so, why not?

8. Do you respect single fathers or not really, and if so why not?

9. How you feel about working with domestic abusers?

10. Do you feel that you are not educated enough, and secretly you feel less than others, if so what is stopping you from going back to school? (be honest with yourself)

11. If you could change something, or anything in your appearance, what would it be, and why?

These questions should help you be honest with yourself, strengthen who you are, and show you areas where you can use some improvement.

ABOUT THE AUTHOR

Sophia Clementina London was born in the Panama Republic of Panama. She is the oldest of six girls and came from a background of strong resilient women. Her great-grandmother was from Calcutta India, and great grandfather was from Jamaica. Sophia holds a Doctorate in International Gender and Human Rights Chaplaincy. She is a Professional Licensed Trauma-Informed Coach, Certified Christian Counselor, Certified Child and Adolescent Trauma Professional, and Community Health Worker Instructor—committed to serving individuals and communities through healing and advocacy. Sophia Clementina is married to an amazing man Jose A London, who regardless of how many shortcomings and traumas from her childhood, loves her unconditionally. Her two daughters, who she calls her world, are successful professionals with many years of serving the community in different capacities. Sophia Clementina has one grandchild who she calls her prince. Family is very important in everything and anything in this world.

Sophia Clementina is the Head Elder in her church and loves the community she belongs to. As a community health worker for more than twenty years, she works with people from all walks of life, in different communities and states to encourage, uplift, counsel, serve, and help all whom she can regardless of race, color, culture, denomination, or beliefs.

Working with immigrants is where her heart is. She came to this country not speaking the language and had to rely on help from family and strangers until she learned the culture and language and now gives back with passion and love. She worked with immigrant families who needed vaccinations for their babies. She worked with the Child and Teen Checkup, making sure the migrants understand why their kids need those vaccinations repeated or new ones to continue going to school in this country.

Her struggles and triumphs in this country stemmed from the desire to give her loved ones a better life.

Sophia Clementina was motivated to write this booklet because she sees new community health workers coming into the profession who are passionate and dedicated to doing their best to give back, uplift, and help their communities. Her hope is to encourage, uplift, and give simple guidance to newcomers who need clear, simple, straightforward counsel.

SCL

www.ingramcontent.com/pod-product-compliance
Lightning Source LLC
LaVergne TN
LVHW022031200926
848481LV00007B/2643
* 9 7 9 8 9 9 8 6 0 1 2 0 0 *